Don't Stress - RELAX
by Wolfgang Matejek

Here's a list of my other books:

How to grow your Therapy Business

How to build a high income business
as a Professional Speaker

Visit my website for great
business related blogs

Table of Contents

1. How does this book work?

I am delighted that you have decided to buy my book and want to thank you. This book is designed to be not just a book but a complete self-help manual about banishing stress and learning to relax.

And the best part of this book is that there is no pressure to start straight away – but to maintain momentum, I suggest that once you start reading, keep going. This will keep you interested and feeding your desire to get started sooner.

How does this book work?

This book contains of a number of subjects that are both self-contained and also part of the programme. You may even want to print the book, so you can add your own notes to the pages as you work through.

My aim with this book is to convey the information you will need to understand about stress and what you can do about it.

As you work your way through the book, at the end of the sections you are required to complete a simple review paper, which will help you to monitor your own progress and to deepen your knowledge.

This way you can be sure that you have understood each section before moving on to the next. Enjoy the journey and relax.

Wolf Matejek (DHP, DCMT, MASC)
Website: www.wmresourcesltd.com

2. Introducing the author

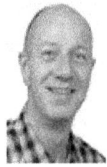

Wolfgang Matejek (*called Wolf by his friends and clients*) is a successful business consultant, trainer, public speaker and part-time therapist. As a business coach and trainer he works with companies world-wide, aiding in the re-structuring of their employee skills and personal development programmes. As a part-time therapist he provides stress management, counselling, coaching, Emotional Freedom Technique (EFT) and hypnotherapy services to private and corporate clients.

Before becoming a self-employed business person, he enjoyed a colourful career in general business management. Having worked in exciting places such as a 5* hotel in Bermuda, running his own restaurant/bar in Germany and also having worked at the world-famous South Bank Arts Centre in London, he played with the idea of a career change.

In 1992, he lost his job as an IT Manager through redundancy. He found himself at cross-roads in his life. This sudden change left him wondering of what to do next. About the same time, a close friend of his fell very ill and suffered from severe depression. And he wanted to help... but didn't know how.

Over the next few years he attended a variety of courses to gain a stronger insight into therapy services and also attained various qualifications to prepare himself for the new adventure as a part time therapist.

In 1994 he qualified as an Aromatherapist. From there he progressed with further studies covering subjects such as counselling, stress management and relaxation therapy. Between his studies he also worked as a freelance business consultant, specialising in the provision of training services as a bespoke systems applications and personal development trainer and consultant.

In 2002, he qualified as a Stress Management Consultant (MASC). He utilises a series of consultations incorporating aspects of stress analysis, relaxation techniques and comprehensive reviews of company productivity channels and coaching of employees and management to perform better in their respective roles. In summer 2006 he finished his qualification as a Hypnotherapist (DHP).

Since then he has been working as an international training consultant, specialising in the employee skills re-distribution and development, delivering workshops and courses in countries around the world.

Now it is your turn to change your own and maybe even other people's lives by learning new stress management skills to enjoy a more rewarding, happier and better life.

Stress is no longer just a 'silent' issue, but is now widely regarded as a modern problem. Some even go as far as to call it a *'modern disease'*.

Instead of reading this book, you could of course make a booking with a complementary therapist to help you with your stress related issues. But their services can vary quite a lot.

To be able to see how you can help yourself or before involving a practitioner, you will need to know the basics about stress also.

So let's begin with your journey to a happier and more fulfilling life.

3. Understanding Stress

Well, no matter how it is put, you have to recognise that there is no universally accepted definition of stress and knowledge of the key definitions that are currently in use. It includes understanding that the stress concept and stress management practice includes issues relating to both causes and effects of stress.

4. Definitions of Stress

Stress arises when individuals perceive that they cannot adequately cope with the demands being made on them or with threats to their well-being. *(R.S. Lazarus (1966). Psychological stress and the coping process. New York: McGraw-Hill)*

Stress, it is argued, can only be sensibly defined as a perceptual phenomenon arising from a comparison between the demand on the person and his or her ability to cope. An imbalance in this mechanism, when coping is important, gives rise to the experience of stress, and to the stress response. *(T. Cox (1978). Stress. Basingstoke: Macmillan Education)*

Stress results from an imbalance between demands and resources. *(R.S. Lazarus and S. Folkman (1984). Stress, Appraisal and Coping. New York: Springer)*

Stress is the psychological, physiological and behavioural response by an individual when they perceive a lack of equilibrium between the demands placed upon them and their ability to meet those demands, which, over a period of time, leads to ill-health. *(S. Palmer (1989). Occupational stress. The Health and Safety Practitioner, 7, (8), 16-18)*

Each one has their own understanding of what stress actually is, but in a nutshell it can be put simply as something like:

Stress occurs when pressure exceeds your perceived ability to cope.

And for the simplicity of this book we shall continue to use this interpretation.

5. Causes and Effects of Stress

Listing the cause of stress is tricky. There can be innumerable stress factors since different individuals react differently to the same stress conditions. Extreme stress situations for an individual may prove to be mild for another, for yet another person the situations might not qualify as stress symptoms at all.

Stress is often termed as a twentieth century syndrome, born out of man's race towards modern progress and its ensuing complexities. For that matter, causes such as a simple flight delay to managing a teenage child at home can put you under stress.

A stress condition can be real or perceived. Yet, our brain reacts the same way to both causes of stress by releasing stress hormones equal to the degree of stress felt. The brain doesn't differentiate between real and imagined stress. It could happen while watching a horror movie or when one is apprehensive of some imminent danger.

It is said that life acts and you react. Our attitude is our reaction to what life hands out to us. A significant amount of stress symptoms can be avoided or aroused by the way we relate to stressors.

Stress is created by what we think rather than by what has actually happened. For instance, handling adopted children, adolescents, academic failures, retirements, tax audits or sudden loss of money needs a relaxed attitude, focused will and preparedness to face the quirks of life positively. Otherwise one tends to feel stressed and reacts in anger and frustration. With a better control of attention one can feel that the world is a more congenial place to live in.

Again, in case of a marital conflict, instead of adopting an accusing and frustrating attitude such as - "*You made my life hell*" or "*You are not meeting my emotional needs,*" the American clinical psychotherapist Willard F. Harley suggests that accepting - "*Yes, we have a problem*", helps clear the clouds. Failure in adopting a realistic attitude to events creates symptoms of depression and aggravates stress situations.

A right attitude can make a resilient person out of us in the face of stressful situations.

Major life events such as a divorce, death, midlife crisis, financial worries, persistent strain of caring for a chronically sick child, nagging health problems or managing a physically or mentally challenged family member can act as potential stressors.

Even conditions such as prolonged unemployment or a sudden lay-off/redundancy from a job can leave you under tremendous stress. One just can't wish away situation. Moreover one has to live through these situations, in the right spirit, to make living a worthwhile experience.

Stress also comes from our personal and social contexts and from our psychological and emotional reactions to such conditioning. Here, our mental and emotional disposition, built over the years, decides whether to accept these situations with a fighting or fleeing spirit. Accordingly, we may either be under harmful influences of stressors or be out of it.

Children and women subjected to mental or physical abuses are known to suffer from tremendous stress symptoms of depression, constant anxiety and burnout. Though anger, fear and other negative emotional reactions are natural and necessary we need to channel them constructively to create a balanced state in our body and mind.

Medically, it has been established that chronic symptoms of anxiety and stress can crumble our body's immune system. Irrespective of the nature of the causes of stress - real or perceived - our subconscious mind reacts with the same body response by releasing stress hormones equal to the degree of our fear, worry or sense of threat.

It brings about changes in the body's biochemical state with extra epinephrine and other adrenal steroids such as hydro-cortisone in the bloodstream. It also induces increased palpitation and blood pressure in the body with mental manifestations such as anger, fear, worry or aggression. In short, stress creates anomalies in our body's homeostasis.

When the extra chemicals in our bloodstream don't get used up or the stress situation persists, it makes our body prone to mental and physical illnesses.

For example, imagine a secretary in an office:

Her boss comes in, angry and furious. He starts blasting the secretary for no apparent reasons. Now, her activated adrenaline cycle would tell her to flee or fight. Her senses become acute, muscles tighten, heartbeats and blood pressure increase and brain activity speeds up.

She would probably like to walk out or alternatively, turn around and punch him in the face. But she does neither; for to do so might mean losing her job.

So what follows?

She burns up a lot of her body energy without achieving anything. At the end of the day she would be left mentally, physically and emotionally exhausted - classic symptoms of anxiety and stress. It can happen to anybody from a high profile businessman to a student, an executive or a homemaker.

All are burning out their energies to defend themselves from their real or perceived causes of stress.

We often remain oblivious to the idea that pets - animals and birds - also suffer from stress. Pets are extremely sensitive to their surroundings and are known to develop emotional bonding with their owners as well as fellow pets. 'Change' triggers stress in animals the same way it triggers stress in humans. Health conditions also affect the pets' psychological state.

Conditions such as illnesses, travel, breeding, separation from owner, shifting, addition or loss of a family member or another household pet, can cause stress in animals. In such cases, pets become extremely bored or show symptoms of severe stress such as fear, anxiety and restlessness.

A bored pet dog would slowly chew, destroy things or move objects in and around the household, eat or drink excessively, and sometimes, even create inflammation conditions like "lick granuloma" (usually an ulcerated area on a dog's wrist or ankle caused by the dog's own incessant licking).

They also tend to bark a lot when they are bored. Stressed-out dogs show signs of shaking, trembling, restlessness and destructiveness. It is just as important to treat boredom, as it is to treat anxiety.

In a challenging situation the brain prepares the body for defensive action - the fight or flight response by releasing stress hormones, namely, cortisone and adrenaline. These hormones raise the blood pressure and the body prepares to react to the situation. With a concrete defensive action (fight response) the stress hormones in the blood get used up, entailing reduced stress effects and symptoms of anxiety.

When we fail to counter a stress situation (flight response) the hormones and chemicals remain unreleased in the blood stream for a long period of time. It results in stress related physical symptoms such as tense muscles, unfocused anxiety, dizziness and rapid heartbeats.

We all encounter various stressors (causes of stress) in everyday life, which can accumulate, if not released. Subsequently, it compels the mind and body to be in an almost constant alarm-state in preparation to fight or flee. This state of accumulated stress can increase the risk of both acute and chronic psychosomatic illnesses and weaken the immune system.

Stress can cause headaches, irritable bowel syndrome, eating disorder, allergies, insomnia, backaches, frequent cold and fatigue to diseases such as hypertension, asthma, diabetes, heart ailments and even cancer. In fact, Sanjay Chugh, a leading Indian psychologist, says that 70% to 90% of adults visit primary care physicians for stress-related problems.

Scary enough?

Just about everybody - men, women, children and even babies - suffer from stress. Relationship demands, chronic health problems, pressure at workplaces, traffic snarls, meeting deadlines, growing-up tensions or a sudden change in lifestyles can trigger stress conditions. People react to it in their own ways.

In some people, stress-induced adverse feelings and anxieties tend to persist and intensify. Learning to understand and manage stress can prevent the counter effects of stress. Methods of coping with stress are aplenty. The most significant or sensible way out is a change in lifestyle.

Relaxation techniques such as meditation, physical exercises, listening to soothing music, deep breathing, various natural and alternative methods, personal growth techniques, visualisation and massage are some of the most effective of the known non-invasive stress busters.

Now that we have explored STRESS in some detail we want to move on and concentrate on how you can make a change to your own life and maybe others around you.

You already understand the basics of stress management and stressor identification, but you will need to spend a bit more time in the background to investigate more details to how you can be more effective in making desired changes.

6. Acknowledgement of Tension

Babies are seen as having the perfect life. No worries, no stress though loved and cherished by everyone. Curious of their new surroundings when awake, but otherwise spending a lot of the time sleeping and relaxing. Aaaah, such bliss…

But is it really…?

Babies are born with two instinctive fears - the fear of fire and loud noise. Either one can cause an immense amount of stress to a baby and even affect their life ahead in a very emotional and psychological way.

Through our lives we accumulate the memories of many different types of experiences, which affect our emotional, physical and mental well-being. Some of those experiences can create mildly tense reactions, whereas others can be quite traumatic. Such traumas can affect our whole life path and cause an immense amount of stress, which over time can cause serious mental and psychological issues.

The human instinct is to protect ourselves whenever there is a danger and this process of self-preservation ingrains itself into our memory. There it forms part of our subconscious but the scars of this tension become imprinted in our physical persona, our body language and behaviour.

This makes our body a store-room of all collected subconscious and conscious material.

The body then memorises such events and creates a pattern of behaviour that will remain with us until we consciously change it. The mind is a fantastic machine that stores and releases information at will, but sometimes some information is so deeply stored that it will need special tools to access that information.

That's because the mind has the ability to cloud over, screen or mask negative information and filter such experiences from re-surfacing.

Learning how to relax the body and mind is a way of re-educating ourselves to finding ways of responding to stress other than the pattern we appear to be locked into. Since most of human behaviour is conditioned, we respond through memory. Bringing with it elements of fear and anticipation, based on previous experiences.

Anticipation of an event in itself can be more stressful than the actual event because the imprint in our memory is so great that the very thought stimulates our body chemistry to release signals of tensions.

This process of conscious change is transformational. It means that you are changing one formation of energy into another formation. Changing what one might call "Bad Habits" into "Good Habits".

All forms of tension are accumulations of blocked energy which over time, have hardened in a more rigid form of behaviour, mental or postural patterns. And it is quite obvious that the more intense or the longer you have held that pattern, the deeper the persona imprint and the harder it will be to change it.

And wherever there is a great deal of tension there is also a great deal of energy. It takes a large amount of energy to maintain tension for a long period of time. This is why people feel a tremendous amount of relief when this tension is released. Relaxation therapy can help with a large number of issues that cause tension in people's bodies and minds, such as:

Insomnia

Impotence

Sciatica

Frozen shoulder

Constipation

IBS (irritable bowel syndrome)

Migraine / Headaches

Tinitus

Asthma

Eczema and Psoriasis

Anxiety attacks

Heart-Palpitations

Shortness of breath

Uncontrollable temper

Irritability

Allergies

PMT

Indigestion

Menopause

Eating disorders such as Bulimia or Anorexia

Obsessive behaviour

Rheumatic pain

Traumatic shock syndrome

Epilepsy

General feeling of stress

7. Conscious Relaxation

Our body is a quite selfish and enjoys nothing more than direct attention. Most of the time the mind works on one or more tasks at the same time as the body does another. We tend to lose touch with our feelings and follow the mind until we suddenly realise we have done something to upset the body.

For example:

We have been thinking about something while twisting our neck too far and cause a discomfort – Pains develop in the shoulder/neck...

Being out of touch with our body and mind creates an imbalance that in itself can cause stress. The practice of conscious relaxation bridges this gap between body and mind to allow the feeling of unity between body and mind in complete self-awareness.

In order to cultivate and nurture deeper awareness and a sense of relaxation we will examine and explore practical knowledge of the way to use our senses.

The senses will enable us to open doors of perception such as hearing, smelling, touching, tasting and conscious control of specific bodily functions, which will help us to balance and harmonise our life experiences while creating a deep sense of well-being.

As you progress through this book you will learn more about the techniques you can use to achieve deep relaxation and body awareness.

8. Therapists a Plenty

The world today is fast living, noisy, smelly and very tiring. Everyone is rushing around, getting things done. Work pressures, personal lives and even spare time activities all house a great deal of stress.

Many people have forgotten how to relax completely. The life balance has tipped and most people find even thinking about relaxation stressful in itself. So they take the easy option in trying to relax by watching TV, smoking, drinking alcohol, taking drugs (illegal and prescription) and/or over-eating.

And those are the most common ways people will take when they are so tense that they do not have the energy or know-how to deal with any problems in any other way. Sometimes medical professionals may tell their patients that they should relax more, but they don't know how to help themselves or where to go for help.

You will need to learn how to change stressful situations and learn how you can achieve and experience a state of deep relaxation. You need to learn how to relax.

You effectively will have to acquire knowledge to be able to use such techniques for yourself. While the need for professional relaxation therapists is growing and people are more willing to see someone who will lead and guide them into that beautiful feeling of total relaxation of body and mind, you can do it all by yourself too.

And with this book you will be able to do just that, giving you the theoretical and practical knowledge and techniques to help yourself and others too.

9. Self Counselling

Before you can successfully analyse and help yourself, it is vital to investigate your health and lifestyle while looking out for other underlying issues.

This can be done through a structured form of open-ended 'self-counselling' questions about your health history and general well-being.

And it is self-evident that by asking yourself questions about your personal issues you may discover things that make you feel stressed. But is the most important stage in which you develop an understanding of the stressors in your life.

Here are some sample questions that may help you along the way to self-discovery:

1. **To whom am I able to turn when I need support and comfort?**
   These may be your best friends or partner. I also could be someone at work that you relate to very well.

2. **Who are the people I should avoid?**
   These may be people at work, who do nothing more but ask questions, yet actually never really listening. Or it could be people who just gossip to other people about your problems.

3. **What can I do for my body to feel healthy?**
   Maybe you tend to smoke too much when stressed, so cutting down would be a lot healthier. Or drink more water, eat more healthily. Go for a walk in the park or start doing some exercise.

4. **What do I need to do or let go off, so I have more time to my own needs?**
   Maybe you do need to say 'NO' once in a while. Or have someone to help you with housework (kids?).

5. **What could I do right now to feel more comfortable?**
   Have a nice hot coco; wear some fluffy slippers or booking yourself an appointment for a great massage at your local beauty salon or spa.

6. **What could I do to distract myself from stressful feelings?**
   Do something that you enjoy doing, such as reading this book or watching a funny movie.

Of course, everyone will respond differently to these questions. And that is the beauty; we are all different in our own ways in doing things.

Ultimately I cannot tell you what the best approach to these questions are, but I know that the aim is for you to learn how to

RELAX!

Other questions you could ask yourself are:

- Am I presently taking any medication?

- What kind and for how long?

- How do I sleep?

- Do I experience any palpitations?

- Am I allergic to anything?

- Do I have sensitive skin?

- Do I have a regular exercise programme?

- Do I experience any physical pain or migraine?

- When tense, do I become: angry, nervous, anxious, etc?

- Are there any colours I like or dislike?

- Which relaxation techniques have I tried before?

- Which ones worked for me?

These are of course just sample questions to help you get an idea and to help you paint a rough picture of your personal lifestyle and highlighting potential issues of concern.

Feel free to expand this list with anything you feel may help you to develop your own style.

10. Review Questions 1

To test your own progress through this book, do answer the following questions honestly. All the answers are somewhere in the book.

Q 1: What is the definition of Stress?

Q 2: What are the causes and effects of stress?

Q 3: What are the side-effects of stress?

Q 4: What illnesses and issues can be treated with relaxation therapy?

Q 5: What is self-counselling?

11. Exercise and Relaxation

Our human body is a machine, designed for physical activity. Over centuries this has helped humans to survive, escape predators and hunt for food. Of course nowadays this is a lot easier. We hunt for food in our local supermarkets and escape predators by hopping on a bus or train or drive away in our own cars.

But this in itself brings a new set of problems...

Try '*hunting for food*' in a supermarket on a Saturday morning...

Hordes of other humans doing the same thing at the same time. Screaming children running amok among the stacks of shelves and parents shouting all over the place for their siblings to calm down. It's a riot! Many people get an overwhelming feeling of anxiety just by the thought of having to mix with those 'food hunters'.

The same happens on the roads. Overcrowded buses and trains. Heavy traffic on the roads causing grid-lock. Once again stress levels rise and so does the road-rage syndrome.

A bleak view of daily life in our world...

Millions of people all over the world jumped on the fitness bandwagon. Gyms all over the place are making record profits from the new health craze. And yes, fitness is vital to our survival. But there has to be a balance.

A relaxed body, by definition, must be one that is free of discomfort and disharmony. And complete relaxation can only be achieved when the body and mind are in harmony, both physically and mentally. While both are interlinked, for the purpose of this book we will treat them separately for closer examination.

Failure to accept these physical requirements and to fulfil them will result in stress and tension and lead to ill health. We also find that certain forms of physical activity provide much more than just physiological efficiency. It will also help us to deal with emotional and intellectual needs to achieve the balance, once we introduce some form of physical activity into our daily life.

There are 2 perspectives to this:

The physical side being able to jump, run, lift, carry things, etc. - as well as the body systems that support life such as breathing, digestion, circulation, nervous systems, etc.

Physical tasks are maintained by the use and control of the skeletal muscular system. Here the muscles work in tandem to achieve results. And every gym can help you to design a personal fitness programme to enable you to maintain a healthy level of fitness.

The other effect on physiology is probably even more important. The whole health and vitality of the individual depends entirely upon the state of the internal support system. No muscular activity is possible without fuel, oxygen, water, trace elements and neural stimulation. The waste products of any muscular efforts have to be removed and eliminated. Not only is the muscular system dependent on these systems, but the whole process of life is supported by a healthy circulatory system.

Should these systems be abused, neglected or dysfunctional for any reason the body will lose large amounts of energy, develop ill health and possibly diseases. Deep relaxation therefore also becomes increasingly more difficult to achieve once the system is in poor condition. The central nervous system is essential to relaxation and once it has been compromised the body will find it difficult to relax.

Exercise programmes will help to maintain the required physical condition for good health, muscular activity and general feeling of well-being. For this reason exercise routines should include a balanced workout of aerobics, anaerobic and stretching elements.

So what is the difference between them?

11.1. Aerobics

Means exercise with air and it is primarily concerned with attaining and maintaining the efficiency of airflow in the body. This covers the areas of respiration and circulation, and the overall desired result is that of a strong heart function. Since both the heart and brain are in need of a regular flow of oxygen, starving either of oxygen will eventually lead to serious defects of the body functions and ultimate death.

Aerobics requires continues activity of at least ½ hour duration. During this exercise routine the heart rate (pulse) must be kept at a level that can be calculated as follows:

Required heart rate = 65% to 75% of 220 minus your age

For example of a person of 40 years of age:

65% x 220 – 40 = approx. 120 beats
75% x 220 – 40 = approx. 135 beats

Calculate your own here:

My age: _____

65% x 220 – 40 = approx. _____ beats

75% x 220 – 40 = approx. _____ beats

To maintain a good level, someone fit would work around the upper level, whereby a 'newbie' to an exercise programme would work closer to the lower level.

11.1.1. Example of Aerobic Exercise

- Running, jogging, fast walking

- Cycling

- Swimming

- Dancing

- Rowing

- Cross-country skiing

It is important to remember that anyone starting out on a new exercise regime should always consult their doctor for advice beforehand and take precautions accordingly.

11.2. Anaerobic

Means that the exercise uses the oxygen already stored in the blood. This pre-stored oxygen in the blood though will run out a lot quicker and therefore the amount of exercise is a lot shorter. But anaerobic exercise is also much more focused on muscular activity and development.

It is more intense but shorter in duration, which takes the form of bursts of effort and recovery in-between, before repeating the process.

11.2.1. Example of Anerobic Exercise

Examples of anaerobic exercise are:

- Weight training

- Interval training

- Some domestic chores like gardening and DIY

11.3. Stretching

Is the warming up process of the muscle groups to enable to body to make good use of the muscular system without causing injury. Stretching exercise should always be done in a controlled and slow motion and without putting any pressure on the muscles to be worked on. Stretching is also often used to relax the body, in such exercises as Yoga.

And it is vital to never overstretch muscles as this can cause damage to muscles, ligaments and tendons. Exercise has to be learned properly to achieve the value of the exercise and to avoid injury. Exercise of any kind should never be undertaken after a meal for at least 1 hour, even longer after a heavy meal. Get a full medical check before starting out on a new exercise regime.

Never exercise when feeling unwell. If you start feeling unwell during any exercise – stop immediately.

Wear the appropriate outerwear as well as the correct footwear for your exercise. Exercising in cold, wet or slippery conditions can be counterproductive. Never exercise when under the influence of alcohol or drugs.

Be aware of your own limitations, so if you had a broken arm a few months ago, it would be crazy to start lifting weights. Listen to your own body – once in tune with it, you will know what is good for it and what is not.

11.4. Exercise and the Effects on the Mind

These are two distinct reactions, one based on the physical reaction to activity (building muscle, be fitter etc.) and the other based on the mental reaction (feeling great, flushed skin etc.).

Some of the effects on the body and brain inter-action caused by exercise are the release of hormones, hyper ventilation, suspension of digestion, changes in blood sugar levels and heart rate. While some of those may actually be desirable, others may be downright dangerous if not properly appreciated.

Hormone release can yield very positive results.

The injection of adrenaline from the adrenal glands on the kidneys is designed to give instant physical energy and mental clarity. Cortisone is also released from the outer part of the adrenal glands to increase the availability of glucose to the muscles and to reduce the reaction to injury.

Endorphins with pain killing and tranquillising properties are released by the brain. These are also being activated in times of stress without any physical activity. Unfortunately if these secretions are not utilised by physical actions, they are accumulated over a period of time and can lead to increased toxicity and disease of the circulatory system.

This build up of hormones is thought to play a major part in certain stress-related diseases. On the other hand these secretions can also help in boosting physical performance and deliver a feeling of well being.

Hyperventilation is the result of too much oxygen in the brain, causing side effects such as light-headedness. In extreme cases it can cause buzzing in the ear, dizziness, tingling sensations in fingers and even fainting. Our body is very sensitive to the levels of oxygen and carbon dioxide in the blood and will react accordingly.

Suspension of the digestive process occurs when the blood supply to the stomach is required by the muscles for other activities. This in turn can cause discomfort and possibly result in stomach cramps, which can be very painful. Even if this extreme reaction is not reached, the mere overloading of the liver and its capacity to regulate the blood sugar levels can give rise to a feeling of heaviness and lethargy and can eventually lead to diabetes.

Overall, exercise can be a very positive action on the whole of the body. Most people refer to exercise as sport, training or physical activity. And it can be broken down further. There is the single person sport or the competitive sport. And lately there has been an upsurge of high adrenaline sport such as bungee jumping, surfing, mountain climbing to name but a few.

Such high level sports provide a huge release of adrenaline to the system that is often followed by deep relaxation. And whichever kind of activity people use, the main importance is to be happy with their chosen form of exercise.

For most, relaxation is only possible when the individual is feeling content and generally happy with themselves. This requires a certain level of physical fitness and a mental and emotional fulfilment, all of which can be obtained though a reasonable amount of regular and sustained physical activity.

11.5. Review Questions 2

Well done. You have now reached the end of the 2nd section of the book. To review your own progress, please answer the following questions honestly. All the answers are somewhere in the book.

Q 1: Describe what a 'relaxed body' means.

Q 2: What is the difference between 'aerobic' and 'anaerobic' exercise?

Q 3: What is important when undertaking any new exercise programme?

Q 4: What is 'hyperventilation'?

11.6. Exercise for the Body

So far we have concentrated our efforts in assessing the benefits of physical exercise for the body. Thus being the stimulation and motivation of the actual muscle groups, limbs, bone structure and respiration that get into motion through assertion of their external strength and power.

But the body is quite selfish. It likes to be pampered a lot more than just being pushed through physical exercise. Looking behind the scenes we find the hidden resource of internal energy. This energy opens up a doorway into an area of exercise and body-mind awareness that utilises a much deeper resource of strength, health and endurance.

This is the approach of working with the subtle energy system that actually governs the balance of our bodily functions with greater emphasis on fluidity, concentration, meditation, prolonged suspension of a posture or movement that promotes an inner harmony of sustained and prolonged well being.

This approach is different as we are actually working from the inside out, rather than from the outside in. Many Eastern cultures have been practicing this approach for many hundreds of years, prime examples being martial arts, particularly Tai Chi, Aikido and Kung Fu.

All of these work with a high level of deep concentration on specific movements that empower and harmonise body and mind simultaneously. Maybe you remember seeing one of those Kung Fu artists using an almost inhuman strength to show off their powers, and it wasn't huge bulks of muscles that help them to achieve such feats like smashing towers of roof tiles or bricks into half.

Yoga is another perfect example of the balancing of the internal subtle energy fields to stabilise, stretch and enliven body structure. The subtle body exercises require some understanding of the invisible energy channels (meridians) on which Chinese medicine is based – the Chakras. In essence, Chakras cover the benefits of directional breathing and other breathing techniques that hold the potential to break down old psycho-physiological patterns and give us new powers.

This type of exercise is seen as a more 'spiritual' practice as it is based upon energy fields that every living creature possesses. And by creating a balance in our lives between stillness and movement, assertion and reception we also create powerful healing energy that reflects itself in the world around us.

11.7. Choosing the Right Exercise

To enable you to find an exercise regime that will work for you and that you also can enjoy, you may want to ask yourself:

- Am I strong boned or soft, muscular or skinny?

- Is my weight and height balance distributed?

You could practice this exercise with members of your own family and friends. To gain an insight into your own assessment, take some time, stand in front of the mirror and complete your own assessment.

You might also want to investigate your spiritual and faith ideologies. And as you take into account all those characteristics and review various options of exercises that would be available, you will find out if you will benefit from yoga or aerobics, or both. Or if you dislike classes you could think about going walking or swimming etc.

You do hold the keys to your own health, well being and happiness. So it would be great if you can make some adjustments to your own life to gain a deeper insight to how you can help yourself or someone you love to live a more enriched life and well being.

Following are some suggestions for exercises:

11.7.1. Subtle Body Exercises

Yoga, Tai Chi can be practiced every day. Benefits are felt even if only 15 minutes are used, but for a more dramatic improvement 2 hours per day will have a profound impact on your daily activities and well being that relaxation becomes a way of life.

11.7.2. Stretching Exercises

These should be performed on a daily basis and cover all major muscle groups. In particular the muscles located at the back of your thigh (hamstrings), the calf muscles, hip joints, lower back, shoulders and neck muscles.

To achieve a safe and fulfilling exercise it is advised to do these exercises after a warm bath/shower and in a warm room.

And if it hurts – **STOP**. Do not force your muscles.

A routine of 15-20 minutes per day should be sufficient, and make sure you keep warm after the exercise.

11.7.3. Aerobic Stretching

A set of 3 days x 20 minutes per week at the heart rate previously calculated is the minimum to achieve results. This exercise regime should achieve a degree of breathlessness but NOT to the point where you will have to stop, as you are too exhausted or feeling dizzy.

Ideally there should be a rest day between sets. In addition to this routine you could include more general activity such as walking briskly or climbing stairs instead of using the lift.

11.7.4. Anaerobic Exercise

Create a routine involving repetitive movement with resistance for the major muscle groups. It would be ideal to do it at least 2 days per week for at least 30 minutes each session, and with rest days in-between.

All those exercises can be performed in the home, or in a 'club' or gym environment. Those who like social interaction or those who need motivation may find a gym environment more fulfilling, whereas those of a shy nature may prefer to start at home on building the confidence to visit a gym.

11.8. Deep Relaxation and Brain Waves

In the everyday waking state the brain manufactures Beta waves, which have the frequency of immediate cognitive response and general recall of appropriate behaviour to a given situation.

When we start to relax by sitting down or perhaps have a bath, Alpha waves are created.

Such Alpha waves slow down the brain activity, yet we remain fully conscious and able to respond physically and psychologically to any given stimuli. In deep sleep Delta waves are produced, that reveals the shutdown of all cognitive behaviour of brain and mind and creates the subconscious state of being.

Deep relaxation is created upon a frequency that we call Theta waves. The Theta wave state is an unusual state of mind as it is not readily available to the body. It has to be created and nurtured with a certain level of mental concentration and focus.

This is a state that combines the function of the brain to identify and correlate physical experience through the senses, while the muscles and complete form of the body is completely relaxed, as if it is in a Delta state.

In this experience you are fully aware of what is going on around you – yet you feel no urge to get involved in any way. This deeply relaxed state defies our habitual response mechanisms by not allowing the mind/body to get involved but instead remain in an observant and open state of being.

In a deeply relaxed state people's sensory mechanisms come down and depending on their psycho/spiritual conditioning or freedom, can reach truly liberating levels of awareness. During the practice of deep relaxation it is vital to stay awake, as Theta waves are lost once we become unconscious. For your own benefit you must ensure that you stay awake by gently reminding yourself of what is going on around you.

After the exercise some people may fall or want to fall into a much-needed sleep. This period of rest will be tremendously refreshing to you, no matter how short this rest may be.

A relaxed person is a happy person...

Relaxation therapy is fundamentally about educating the mind and body to find new ways to deal with stress and other negative patterns we are locked into. So remaining conscious through the learning process is vital to help you to change negative aspects of life into positive experiences.

Next you will need to do some homework in preparing for your progressive relaxation exercise. Yes, you need to do some recording work.

Ouch, I hear you say. Never done that before? Well, you could also get some ready-made relaxation CDs from the internet, or create your own.

Let me tell you how you can create your own though..., just in case...

11.8.1. Create your own Progressive Relaxation Recordings

If you need some great relaxing background music you can get by visiting http://www.ambient-mixer.com/

Their sounds are free and the site allows you to create your own sound mix. While these relaxing sound waves are great, we are looking to create your own 'bespoke' progressive relaxation recording, since this will help you achieve a much deeper relaxation.

There are a few things you will need to achieve this:

1. A progressive relaxation script to use (provided on the following pages)

2. Some way to record your voice when reading the script aloud (MP3 recorder, PC with microphone)

3. A quiet place to do the recording (turn off the phone, send the kids out to play)

I have provided you with a complete progressive relaxation script you can use. Plus there are additional scripts for your use later in the book.

To record your voice (or someone else doing it for you), you will need to have some way to record this. If you have an MP3 player or a laptop PC with a microphone then you are half-way there.

Recording on an MP3 player is a simple as 'press record' and start to read the script slowly and calmly.
If you are planning to record it on your laptop/PC, then you will need some software to translate your spoken words into sound.

The best and FREE software to do this is called Audacity, which you can download from http://www.audacity.com

Then it's just a matter of installing the software, plugging in your headset microphone and to start recording. The end result can then be saved as an MP3 file to copy and listen to on your phone or MP3 player. You could also burn this file onto CD if you wish.

Alternatively you can buy ready-made CD's on the internet, or email me to create one for you at reasonable cost.

Here are some tips to observe when creating your own relaxation recording:

· Ensure the tone of your voice is calm and confident.

- The speed of your reading the script – Take your time, read it slowly, don't rush. It is actually more beneficial when it is slow rather than too fast.

- The inflection in your voice should be true and realistic. Don't drone on, but also don't overdo it.

- Put some emotion into your voice.

- Remember that the overall effect you wish to create is one of **RELAXATION.**

If you are using background relaxation music, make sure it is not too loud as to drown out your words!

11.8.2. Progressive Relaxation Script for your recording

In the previous section you have learned how to create your own recording. Now that you know how and what to do, you need to have the material to record.

Here are the instructions:

Using the same pattern of breath throughout the sequence as is described in Step 1 below, taking time to relax and reflect on the inner rhythms of the heart and breath after one has exhaled and relaxed the muscle. Take it slowly, giving time for the registering of enjoyment in the experience.

Note: Do not read out the instructions written in *italic letters while recording your personal recording*!!!

The relaxation script:

Step 1: Inhale deeply though the nose, point the toes downwards, tensing the feet and holding the breath tighter and tighter to the slow count of 5…

Pursing the lips slowly blow air out letting the feet fall open and relax.

Wait approximately 30 seconds before moving onto step 2.

Use this period of time to help you achieve and maintain inner focus of the relaxation response and body awareness. It is most effective to close the eyes and focus on each muscle as one goes through the process.

Now slowly continue to read out each instruction, taking short breaks between each one...

- Inhale and flex the feet upwards – exhale etc.

- Inhale and pull up the left knee and thigh muscles

- Exhale and lower the knee in time with your breath and relax

- Inhale and pull up the right knee and thigh muscles

- Exhale and lower the knee in time with your breath and relax

- Inhale and squeeze the buttocks

- Inhale and extend the abdomen – exhale and draw abdominal muscles inward

- Inhale into upper lungs and lift the chest

- Inhale and raise shoulders to the ears – exhale and pull arm down, spanning fingers and stretching arms

- Inhale and flex both arms at elbow, tensing deltoid muscles – exhale etc.

- Inhale and lift head a few inches off the floor – exhale etc.

- Inhale and raise the eyebrows – exhale etc.

- Inhale and tighten and scrunch up the whole face and eyes – exhale etc.

- Inhale and open the mouth and jaw wide – and as one exhale let out an AAAHHH sound

During these stages help yourself to remain focused on your body/mind. Remind yourself of how good it feels to relax and keep yourself from falling asleep.

Once the recording is completed, then this technique takes about 15-20 minutes to complete. It can best be practised horizontally in bed, on the floor or if you prefer in a comfy chair. But horizontally is best.

There are a huge selection of relaxation music tracks available on the market. You may order relaxation CD's from the internet, or email me to create your own bespoke version for you at reasonable cost.

If you were using a music track it would be beneficial to wear a light set of headphones and loose fitting clothes while doing the exercise.

If you do not use an mp3 track it is advised to perform this exercise in a relatively quiet environment, and warm and loose clothes should also be worn. A tracksuit may be just fine.

11.8.3. Review Questions 3

You seem to be moving through the book very nicely. By now you already have acquired some great skills and understanding of stress management. And it's testing time again.

To review your own progress, please answer the following questions honestly. All the answers are somewhere in this book.

Q 1: How would you choose the right exercise programme for yourself?

Q 2: What are 'subtle' exercises?

Q 3: What is 'anaerobic' exercise?

Q 4: Please explain what 'Alpha-waves' and 'Beta-waves' are.

Q 5: When are 'Delta-waves' created?

11.9. Deep Relaxation and Sleep

Sleep is the most natural and instinctive remedy to balance and replenish used energy. No one needs to be trained of how to fall asleep and to experience this ultimate relaxation. The body naturally lets us know when it needs to shut down certain functions to re-charge its resources.

Yet there are cases where people have difficulties going to sleep and are being deprived of this ultimate re-charge of the system. Over prolonged periods of time this sleep deprivation can cause havoc with our body. It can cause mental instability, frustration, stress and even hallucinations. Sleep clinics the world over are still investigating this most mysterious phenomena we posses.

Generally speaking though, sleep is a natural process whereby vital neuro-chemicals are released through the brain that nourish and rebuild our bodily functions, enabling us to maintain a balanced awareness of our participation in the physical, active world.

It is this natural process of actually falling asleep that is so vital to receiving the benefits of this state. Some people are being helped to sleep by using drugs. But this isn't actually the same as sleeping, as one is medically de-sensitised to the tensions that need to be released and instead is blacking out events rather than allowing the body to go through its process of 'letting go' naturally.

This is of course where the practice of relaxation techniques comes in as a bridge between the two world of wakefulness and sleep, when we cannot naturally fall asleep due to the excessive build up of tension that prevents the natural process form happening. Once again we see the need to re-educate the body/mind of its potential for the transformation of negative energy into positive.

11.9.1. Levels or Types of Sleep

Researches into the phenomena of sleep have used electroencephalographs (EEG) to discover what happens in the sleep state. By using this equipment, electrical brain activity has shown that 2 types of sleep patterns occur – named 'orthodox' and 'paradoxical'.

Orthodox sleep has been divided into 4 separate levels of brain activity, the first being a very light state during which one can be awoken easily, yet brain waves have begun to slow down as have the pulse and breathing.

The 2nd and 3rd stages prove to be of special interest to a relaxation therapist as what occurs is a natural process of progressive relaxation during which the muscles relax more deeply and the heart rate and breathing continue to slow down and become more rhythmic.

The 4th level reveals a state of very deep sleep that is usually unconscious, where the brain generates the long and slow Delta waves, characteristic to the reduction in mental activity.

11.9.2. The Effects and Benefits of Orthodox Sleep

As the body and mind start to slow down in the process of orthodox sleep, the body cells begin to divide at a much faster rate, providing the body with a well-needed opportunity to refresh and replenish itself.

Growth hormones are also released into the blood stream during the deepest levels of orthodox sleep. And this deep level of orthodox sleep is required for the body to regenerate itself.

11.9.3. Paradoxical sleep

The most mysterious of all sleep levels, as it relates to our dream state – whether or not we remember the dreams we have had. In this state our brain waves move rapidly, which sometimes can be observed through REM (Rapid Eye Movement), an increased heart rate, physical movements during the sleep and an increase in our blood pressure.

Even though there are signs of inner activity, our muscles are generally more relaxed than in a deep, orthodox sleep state. Dream analysis, interpretations and the understanding of what happens during the dream stage is assumed to be a reflection of our deeper feelings and thoughts, a re-living of an experience and perhaps helps us to sort out 'unfinished business'.

11.9.4. Benefits of Paradoxical Sleep

Orthodox sleep helps the body to re-generate itself, whereas the paradoxical sleep helps the brain to re-balance our mental harmony. People, who awaken frequently during their sleep, often feel washed out and un-rested.

This is because the 90-minute cycle of deep rest and inner mental activity (paradoxical and orthodox sleep) is interrupted.

11.9.5. Sleep Requirements

As we grow older, our requirement for sleep decreases quite extensively. As babies we required about 16 hours sleep per day, reducing gradually to level out during adulthood to between 6 to 10 hours. In older age we get by with just about 6 hours, which seem to be enough as the body reduces the physical and mental demands placed upon us.

Research also has shown that people who meditate regularly do require less sleep, as they manage their relaxation through meditation and thereby reducing their stress levels accordingly.

Absence of a general relaxed attitude in our waking state can either cause us to sleep too much which can make us lethargic, or to not be able to unwind at all, making us hyper. Both of these symptoms can be treated through the practice of relaxation techniques.

11.10. Meditation Techniques

With so many forms of meditation around, it would go beyond the scope of this book to describe each of them. But if you want to find out more, you can visit the following site: http://www.meditationsociety.com/intro.html or do a general search on any of the internet search engines and directories.

But for the simplicity of this book we look at the main process used in all forms of meditation, which is called **Attention**.

Over the last 20 years or so, the Western world has become more and more focused on the philosophies of the East and the powerful effects of meditation on our psychology and behaviour. Meditation began to be viewed not only in the context of a particular spiritual or religious belief, but as a tool for developing awareness and peace of mind and body.

Meditation is essentially a mental exercise of deliberately focusing on a specific sound, object or mental process. And as the mind absorbs this given point of focus, one can experience a sense of calm and rest. And as meditation is regarded as purely experimental, the only way to explore and feel its effects is to experience it in practice.

And as I already said, there are too many different techniques, names, origins and philosophies to cover in this book. But you may want to at least try some out for yourself, so that you are able to ascertain if meditation is for you.

11.10.1. Benefits of Meditation

Meditation has been proven to help reduce the heart rate, calming the mind and nervous system as well as reducing physiological arousal. The breathing reduces substantially which is an important aspect in the revealing of insights into psychological and emotional conditioning.

And with the slowing down of these functions our ability to copy with pressure increases. Most illnesses and diseases are fed by anxiety and fear around it. Meditation can help recovery from these traumas through the development of a more relaxed relationship with body, our mind and ourselves.

For example, when a person is anxious, frightened, agitated, or distracted, the breath tends to get shallow, rapid, and uneven. On the other hand, when the mind is calm, focused, and composed, the breath is slow, deep, and regular. Focusing the mind on the continuous rhythm of inhalation and exhalation provides a natural object of meditation.

As you focus your awareness on the breath, your mind becomes absorbed in the rhythm of inhalation and exhalation. As a result, your breathing will become slower and deeper, and the mind becomes more tranquil and aware.

11.10.2. When to Practice Meditation

Meditation is best practiced at the beginning and the end of the day. In this way you are opening and closing your conscious mind for the day ahead and the end of the day.

I estimate a minimum of 15 minutes to an hour to be sufficient, and it would be helpful to do so in a quiet space, indoors or out. It sometimes helps to set up a meditating room/area with special pictures, icons or even burning incense sticks and soothing music in order to infuse the atmosphere with spiritual energy.

In the East, the cross-legged postures, with head and back in vertical line, are considered ideal for meditation. In the classic Lotus posture, when the legs are crossed with the feet on the thighs, right feeling of poised sitting for meditation is imparted.

These postures are difficult and even painful at first for those who are not familiar with them. For such inexperienced individuals, it may be easier to keep their spine straight by sitting on a well-backed chair or sit on a meditation stool.

It is important to keep the body as still as possible, so rest your hands consciously on the thighs with the thumb and forefinger touching in circles.

11.10.3. Preparing to Meditate

As we are concentrating on the breath technique we are starting as follows:

- Inhale slowly and deeply though the nose
- Hold the breath for around 6 seconds
- Purse the lips and exhale a little breath at a time through the mouth; pausing between each short exhalation for about a second until you are empty of breath
- Pause for 5 seconds
- Repeat the procedure 5 more times
- Our breathing is the only "involuntary" function we can voluntarily control. Breath carries life energy and substance in our existence. And without breath, there would be no 'Us'.

Now let's carry on with the process:

- Let's relax the body by concentrating on each part in turn, allowing the stress in that area to fall away.

- Spend two to five minutes on this.
- Continue to concentrate on the breath, and simply watch it come and go.
- Allow your breathing to become regular and a little deeper, but don't force anything.
- If your mind wanders off in any direction, gently bring it back to an awareness of each breath you take.
- Spend a few minutes just 'watching' the air going into your nose, and then out through the mouth. Try to maintain this simple awareness.
- Breath comes in, and breath goes out.
- Now let your attention focus on the sensations you can feel at the end of your nose or your lips as the air passes through on it's way in and out.
- Relax. Simply 'watch'.

When you are ready, come out of the meditation by gradually becoming aware of your surroundings, and open your eyes. Stretch out. If it helps, put your hands on the floor for a short time as a way of 'coming back to earth'.

11.10.4. Review Questions 4

To test your own progress, please answer the following questions honestly. All the answers are somewhere in the book.

Q 1: What are possible negative effects of sleep deprivation?

Q 2: How can relaxation help in cases of sleep deprivation?

Q 3: Describe the term 'orthodox sleep'.

Q 4: What is paradoxical sleep?

Q 5: What are the average sleep requirements for an adult?

Q 6: What is meditation?

Q 7: What are the benefits of meditation?

11.11. Using Colour for Deep Relaxation

Colour healing, light therapy and chromo therapy are all terms used interchangeably with Colour Therapy, which is a set of principles used to create harmonious colour and colour combinations for healing. Colour therapy (chromo therapy) helps improve and balance emotional state when gaze at selected colours and absorb their energy.

A therapist trained in colour therapy uses colour to balance energy wherever our bodies are lacking, be it physical, emotional, spiritual, or mental.

The body tells us the truth about how we feel and shows us that there is an imbalance in our physiology. Most of the time, we do not pay attention to our body because the pain of feeling and knowing may be too much. The eidetic-mans carefully and compassionately shows us what is needed through images to heal and activate the body and mind toward better health.

Build a collection of coloured cards so that at times to time you can select a colour, focus on it, and restore yourself to a balanced state. Gaze at the colour for as long as you feel you need to. Depending on the severity of the imbalance in your energy, it may take as long as one minutes before a sense of irritation begins to be felt as the saturation point for a colour's energy is reached.

Colour experience provides the opportunity to discover for yourself, the impact colours can have on well-being. The need for a particular colour's energy seems to differ from day to day or even from hour to hour.

When you absorb colour energy it go, via the nervous, to the part of the body that needs it. Each body has its own optimum state of well-being and is constantly seeking ways to maintain or restore a balanced state. Utilizing colour is one way you can help yourself to harmony!

Waveforms of light are expressed in light frequencies called nanometers. For example, red is expressed as 660 nanometer. White light is expressed as a compendium of all the visible light frequencies, which include red, orange, yellow, green, blue and violet.

A great website covering this hugely interesting subject can be found at
http://www.colourtherapyhealing.com

11.11.1. Interpretation of the Colours

Black

This colour is comforting, protective and mysterious. It is associated with silence, the infinite, and the feminine life force-passive, uncharted and mysterious. Black can also prevent us from growing and changing. We often cloak ourselves in black to hide from the world.

White

The colour of ultimate purity is white. It is an all-around colour of protection, bringing peace and comfort, alleviating emotional shock and despair, and helping inner cleansing of emotions, thoughts, and spirit. If you need time and space to reflect on your life, white can give you a freedom, and uncluttered openness. Too much white, however, can be cold and isolating.

Blue

Blue is a cool, calming colour and is associated with a higher part of the mind than yellow. It represents the night, so it makes us feel calm and relaxed as if we are being soothed by the deep blue of the night sky.

Light and soft blue, make us feel quiet and protected from all the bustle and activity of the day, and alleviates insomnia. Blue inspires mental control, clarity, and creativity. Midnight blue has a strong sedative effect on the mind, allowing us to connect to our intuitive and feminine side. Too much dark blue however can be depressing.

Violets and Purple

These have a deep effect on the psyche and have been used in psychiatric care to help calm and pacify patients suffering from a number of mental disorders and nervous disorders. These colours balance the mind and help transform obsessions and fears. Violet and purple are colours of transformation at a very deep level, bringing peace and combating fear and shock.

They have a cleansing effect in emotional disturbances. They are also connected with artistic and musical impulses, mystery, and sensitivity to beauty and high ideals, stimulating creativity, inspiration, sensitivity, spirituality and compassion.

Violet can exert strong psychic influences, however, and a person attracted by it has to guard against living in a fantasy world. Purple is associated with psychic protection.

Greens

Green has a strong affinity with nature, helping us connect with empathy to others and the natural world. We instinctively seek it out when under stress or experiencing emotional trauma. It creates a feeling of comfort, laziness and relaxation, calmness, and space, lessening stress, balancing and soothing the emotions. Dark green represents the onset of death and is non-descript, unassertive, a negation of love and joy.

Lime green and olive green can have a detrimental effect on both physical and emotional health since sickly yellow and green are associated with the emotions of envy, resentment, and possessiveness.

Yellows and Gold

Yellow is also a happy, bright, and uplifting colour, a celebration of sunny days. It is associated with the intellectual side of the mind, and the expression of thoughts. It therefore aids the powers of discernment and discrimination, memory and clear thinking, decision-making and good judgment.

It also helps good organisation, assimilation of new ideas, and the ability to see different points of view. It builds self-confidence and encourages an optimistic attitude. Conversely, dull yellow can be the colour of fear.

Like yellow, gold is associated with the sun, and therefore related to abundance and power, higher ideals, wisdom and understanding. It is mentally revitalising, energizing and inspiring, and helpful for fear, uncertainty, and lack of interest. Pale gold is excellent for depression and sharpens the mind.

Red

Red is a powerful colour that has always been associated with vitality and ambition. It can help overcome negative thoughts. However, it is also associated with anger; if we have too much red in our system, or around us, we may feel irritable, impatient, and uncomfortable.

Orange

Orange is a joyous colour. It frees and releases emotions and alleviates feelings of self-pity, lack of self worth, and unwillingness to forgive. It stimulates the mind, renewing interest in life. It is a wonderful anti-depressant and lifts the spirits. Apricot and Peach are good for nervous exhaustion.

Pink

Pink is emotionally soothing and calming, and gives a feeling of gentle warmth and nurturing. It lessons feelings of irritation and aggression, surrounding us with a sense of love and protection. It also alleviates loneliness, despondency, over sensitivity, and vulnerability. While red relates to sexuality, pink is associated with unselfish love.

Colour all around...

Now you can see how important colours are in our daily lives. They have incredible powers on our well-being and overall mental attitude.

Colours also are being used extensively to create moods and to encourage certain customer behaviour and buying instinct. This is especially important in sales of perfume, clothes and home furnishings.

I hope this short colour introduction helps you to think of the ideal colours for your home and even on the clothes you wear.

You may also think of changing light bulb colours to change the ambiance of your rooms, depending on the mood you wish to create. To change the light colour you could consider so called Lighting Gels, which are used in theatres to change the lighting colour, as changing bulbs would be too cumbersome and limiting. A website that could help you is http://www.formatt.co.uk/gels/default.asp

And as you continue your progress through this book you will find that the information on colours also helps with the area of visualisation.

11.11.2. Review Questions 5

To test your own progress, please answer the following questions honestly. All the answers are somewhere in this book.

Q 1: What are the benefits of colour therapy?

Q 2: How does colour impact on people?

Q 3: What are the benefits of the colour 'white'?

Q 4: What are the dangers of too much 'red'?

Q 5: Which colour is associated with psychics?

Q 6: What are the benefits of the colour 'green'?

Q 7: What would be a suitable colour for a bedroom, and why?

11.12. Visualisation through Imagination

The influence of imagination over actual experiences can have a very powerful effect. People usually never realise how much imagination controls of our thoughts and actions. The mind is so easily underestimated. But once we learn how to manipulate it, we can achieve great things.

Visualisation takes place when the mind reproduces an image, even though no source for the image is present for the eyes to see. Researchers have questioned whether mental imagery created through visualisation is closely linked to the same processes the brain uses when images are perceived by the eyes. In some cases, the answer appears to be "Yes."

A picture is worth a thousand words.

We've all heard that saying before! This has never been truer than in the case of using Visualisation. Visualisation is an excellent tool to deal with the stresses and negatives in your life. Visualisation, a meditation technique, uses pictures or imagery to balance the brain and boost our body back to total health.

The brain is divided into two sides - our left logical side and our right creative side. Most of our life is spent using the left, logical side of the brain. By using visualisation we yield to our right creative side and produce a balance of the brain. This balance of the brain aids the natural healing processes of the mind and body and opens us up to change and renewal.

Visualisation uses imagery to change your emotions, which changes your feelings, which then turns into physical sensation that can relieve or eliminate symptoms.

The mental form of the mind is emotion and emotion produces feelings. The body's physical form is sensation. When we get an emotion it produces a feeling that turns into a physical sensation. (e.g. Watch a scary movie, get frightened, get goose bumps.)

Visualisation provides positive images for the mind that change your emotions that produce a feeling, which turns into a sensation. That's how you access your mind-body connection.

Remember, YOU ARE WHAT YOU THINK!   SO...THINK POSITIVE!

It has been proven that negative emotions lower our immune system and keeps us bogged down mentally. Having negative emotions delays and stops us from reaching our goals and actually inhibits the brain in accomplishing what we want.

A positive emotion actually boosts the immune system and helps the brain to work in a balanced mode, which is conducive to change.

11.13. How do you keep a positive Balance to your Brain?

1. Can't Keep Positive if you try to control situations.

This uses the left-brain and puts right side out of balance and actually creates a Paradox or Contradiction in the brain. Have you ever wanted something so much that it doesn't happen? Then when you don't want it, it happens?

That's because trying to control a situation makes your goals rigid and actually inhibits the mind-body connection in accomplishing what you want.

2. Can't keep positive if you SET expectations, significance, attitudes or feelings on what we want.

Like control, these make our goals rigid and actually prevent you from accomplishing what you want.

3. Can't Keep Positive if you worry about what other people think.

We have to recognise who we are and accept ourselves. Every one of us is special and has special gifts. It's our choice whether we use them or not.

4. Can't keep positive if you confuse happiness with fulfilment of desires.

Wanting is natural in life but the idea that we can't be happy unless we satisfy a certain desire is not!

5. Can't keep Positive if you insist on being right.

or what I call "My Way is the Only Right Way". The insistence on always being right shows a small view of the world. It makes you feel safe but stops communication, awareness of new changes and stops the ability of choice and usually relies on anger and blame to create a sense of your own independence, but it all it really does is cut you off from Positive Thought.

6. Can't Keep Positive if you use Rationalisation.

This is where you assemble an explanation to conform to your perspective - But it has no foundation! You falsely attribute to others your own way of thinking, feeling and acting. No two people are alike, so this strategy fails.

When your head and heart can't come together it's called rationalisation.

7. Can't Keep Positive if you use I SHOULD.

This is usually based on false social beliefs (e.g., wearing a particular brand of clothing) that keep us plunged into negative feelings not positive ones.

8. Can't keep positive if you live in the Past or the Future.

This keeps your mind fragmented and stops you from accomplishing what you want. You can't do anything about the past - it s over. You can' t do anything about the future because there are too many variables that could happen. So you have to learn to focus on the moment. Concentrating on the moment allows you to accept change easier and enjoy each moment of life.

You need to forget the past that is stopping us from what we want to accomplish and learn to deal with NOW in THIS MOMENT. By living in the moment life flows. You then set up loose goals, put the intention of what you want to accomplish to work and then let any attachment to the outcome go so it CAN be accomplished.

Remember to focus on the <u>Intention</u> and not the results.

11.13.1. What is Intention?

Let's use the example of eliminating some stress in your life:

1. **Intention is NOT** trying to control the outcome, like thinking, "I WILL be stress-free!"

2. **Intention is NOT** negative thinking, like thinking, "I'll never be stress free!"

3. **Intention is NOT** disillusionment, like thinking, "There's nothing I can do about this."

4. **Intention is NOT** the ego, like thinking, "I can make myself be stress free."

5. **Intention is NOT** rationalisation or setting up expectations or rigid goals like "If I exercise by next week I'll be stress free."

Intention is to feel, trust and know that being stress-free is being accomplished!

Can it be that simple?

Yes, if we get rid of the negative programming in our lives. Remember our body, mind and spirit are working 24 hrs a day, 365 days a year to manifest what we want to make us joyful and happy.

Visualisation helps put INTENTION to work.

So far this sounds very appealing. But how do I help myself in this person centred process?

There is a fantastic way to accomplish this, which is called: *VISUALISATION*.

11.14. Guided Visualisation

You are effectively setting out to experience the visual world you use to relax. But of course you need to have some preparation at hand before you can proceed with this particular approach.

Firstly, and most importantly you will need to know from within yourself which visual experience will actually help you to relax rather than to scare you or make you anxious.

For example:

You may have grown up in the country, while living in a big house near a river. The weather in the country during the summer created lots of thunderstorms and as a child you may have been terrified of lightning and the loud thunder claps and rumbles. Or you may never have learned to swim...

If your guided visualisation would include any references to the above issues of 'storms', 'rivers/water', and/or 'swimming' – it would create a high level of anxiety in yourself rather than helping you to relax. It is imperative to ensure that you have covered any negative experiences before setting out to compose your guided visualisation script.

The other things that may help you would be a soothing relaxation music track, which is highly effective in enriching your visualisation experience. The rhythm and pitch of your voice is also a vital key in establishing a rapport with your mental receptivity to what you are saying.

Let your voice sound full and deep, with regular breathing intervals, freeing any tension from your voice. If you speak too fast or too high, you will not give yourself enough space to develop the images in your mind or get in touch with your inner feelings.

Since this is a guided 'tour', enjoy this journey.

Be sensitive to the picture you are 'painting' in your mind. You MUST aim to give yourself the feeling and REAL sense of actually being there. And the more evocative and powerful the images, the more powerful they are in triggering the physiological response of relaxation and well-being.

And such visualisation recordings can once again be recorded by yourself, bought readily on the internet or provided by me if you wish.

Once the recording is done, it's time to test it out.

Make sure that you can sit in a comfortable chair or maybe even lie down on a comfortable couch. The room should be semi-dark and warm, and a soft scent of lavender will aid relaxation.

Let's have a look at a visualisation sample script I have provided for you.

11.14.1. Forest Walk Script

Visualize yourself now in a beautiful forest…

It's a crisp autumn day and the dappling sun reflects upon a gurgling stream that runs along the edge of the forest.

You tread carefully into the forest, over the crackling red and golden leaves and broken twigs;

Pine cones are scattered across the ground - a squirrel runs up a tree - you watch the speed with which it moves, swiftly up and through the branches until you lose sight of it.

It's a very peaceful life here in this forest - you notice clusters of bluebells and soft green moss.

And the deeper into the forest you venture, the deeper into relaxation you fall - you're falling deeply into a calm and tranquil feeling.

Watch a leaf falling from a tree as it dances and twirls in the air, before fluttering slowly down to rest with the others.

You pause for a while and rest against an old oak tree.

You can feel the rough bark of the tree against your fingertips - smell the earthy ground and soft leaf mould - fairy rings of toadstools or mushrooms scattered here and there, and even as you're resting here against the rough bark of the tree, you can feel a deep sense of peacefulness in this beautiful place.

And this deep sense of peacefulness is growing and developing within you - its growing stronger and stronger each and every day.

Each and every day you are growing stronger and stronger - as strong as an old oak tree, stronger and stronger each and every day.

Because now - your body knows how to relax.

In the appendices you find further samples of guided visualisation scripts (hypnosis scripts), which will give you an idea of how to 'paint' with words. And once again you can use those samples to help you to create your own.

And with other parts in this book, you are welcome to share all your new knowledge to practice on friends and family to build your own experience.

11.14.2. Review Questions 6

To test your own progress, please answer the following questions honestly. All the answers are somewhere in the training materials.

Q 1: What is visualisation?

Q 2: Describe 'intention'.

Q 3: What is a guided visualisation?

Q 4: Do write your own guided visualisation script of either:

      - A walk in the park

      - A walk on the beach

      - A winter's day

12. Appendices

A-Z progressive relaxation script

Country-walk hypnosis script

Progressive muscle relaxation script

How to be calm in a stressful situation

How to Create A Home Spa Experience Without
Spending A Fortune

How to de-stress yourself

How to have a day of relaxation (for women)

How to relax

12.1. A to Z for Relaxation

Finding a comfortable place to sit or recline...just taking a few deep breaths...in...and out....in...and out...

Allowing yourself to relax all over...letting all of your muscles and all of your tendons go loose....go limp...go heavy...

Today....we're going to relax....because...you're entering into hypnosis today with the intention of learning to relax...to let go of stress, anxiety and anger....to just...be...at peace...enjoying life...

So as you recline...allowing yourself to let go...perhaps we can begin going through the alphabet...and each letter that I say...can take you deeper...maybe ten...maybe fifteen...maybe even twenty times deeper than you've ever been before...

Beginning with **A**....which stands for air...try to resist breathing in deeply....try to resist noticing how relaxing that breathing in can be...

B...is for breath...because as you breath...you can relax, breathing in the good air, and breathing out the bad...

C is the English equivalent for the Greek letter gamma...which is like a game...like those little things in life...are a game...they're trifling and unimportant...and you can just let them go...

As you relax even deeper...

D...is for dancing...such a joyful carefree activity...you can dance through life...enjoying every moment...and leaving dull care behind...

E... is for ethereal...in the realm of ether - just...air...blowing in the breeze...in the wind...

F... is for fun...because, you know, people are able to have fun each and every day...

G... is for grand...you may have already started to notice that your life is grand...and so far above the little things...

As you find yourself going deeper...

H... is for heart - people are able to live life listening to their heart...with calm compassion...such peaceful...calm...compassion...

I...like your eyes...can see...see past the smoke...see what's really going on...appreciate...what's going on past, above, beyond the little things...

J... is for joke...remembering the feeling you get as you realize and appreciate...how it feels...to enjoy a joke...

K... is for karma...people are able to notice your good karma...as you display your calm happiness...

L... is for love...that wonderful feeling that is in your heart...each and every day...that influences how you interact with kind calm compassion towards others...

M... is for malleable...like gold...gold, you know, can adapt...it can bend....its malleable...adjusting to whatever the situation is...just like you...can adjust, when the situation arises...

N... is for the new energy and ideas that you carry with you on a daily basis...

As you become more - perhaps fifteen, perhaps twenty...maybe even thirty or forty times more relaxed...

O... is for others - a person may know that they can change themselves...and that others cannot destroy your peaceful sense of wellbeing...

P... is for purpose - you have a purpose...you know your purpose...and it guides you...very peacefully...very pleasantly...

Q... is for Quixotic - your life is your own...you create your own world...you choose what it is for you...

R... is for Relaxation- letting go of all that troubles you

S... is for Success - a person may not know that it is easy to achieve success in self-control...

T... is for truth....I wonder if you've already started to notice that, the truth is, that you're in complete control...

U... is for utilize...your assets - you can utilize all of your assets - because you control them...they are what you make them...

V... is for victory....You may be aware of your victory over stress as you notice how easy it is to be in control...

W... is for wind....as your worries and annoyances can blow away in the wind...just drifting off...into nowhere...

X... is for excitement....one of the things you're really going to love about being in control is that you can be so excited about all of your wonderful accomplishments...

Y... is for youth....you can always carry youthful joy around as your go about your life...

As your relax more....

Perhaps noticing the **Z**'s as they fill a comic bubble...indicating that a character is asleep...maybe...in a state of hypnotic relaxation...

12.2. Country Walk Hypnosis Script

I want to take you on a magical journey inside yourself - to a beautiful place outside in nature. And it's a lovely warm summer's day and the sun is shining down on you.

You're strolling along a country path - ambling aimlessly - just enjoying the wonderful view - the rolling green hills and the wild plant life - the hedgerows and tress - and all the beautiful colours in nature. The trees are swaying gently in the warm summer breeze - and the call of a songbird reaches your ears.

It's a peaceful place and you feel so calm and so tranquil. To the left of you is a small wooded area and further on is a farmhouse and outbuildings - to your right is a field of corn - and the country air smells so fresh - and so invigorating.

Although your body is moving - you feel still - and it's a beautiful feeling - to be so relaxed - and calm and at peace with nature.

As you pass by the wooded area you see another path leading off to your left and you turn the corner and continue your journey.

And there you notice a slow flowing stream and the sound of the water lulls you deeper into a feeling of awe and reverence - you're walking along the bank of the stream - and feeling quite tired after this walk - so you decide to lie down on the bank and enjoy the quietness of this summer afternoon.

As you lie back - you can feel the warmth of the sun on your body - it's as though that sunlight is being absorbed into every cell - every consciousness - every atom of your body - it's good to be so relaxed - and quite perfect to be here right now.

And here - in your perfect place - you can allow your mind to drift - and to wander back - to another time in your life - when you felt so good - a special time - when you did something right - something that made you feel confident and so certain of your own abilities - remember that time now as the memory springs to mind.

I'll be quiet for a while to allow you to really enjoy this memory again - in rich detail - almost as though you're back there - reliving it all over again.

(Pause)

Now bring your attention back to my voice whilst holding those wonderful feelings in your mind - and take a deep breath - a very deep breath - and then sigh - slowly - allowing the air from your mouth - and I want you to see a fluffy white cloud floating above you - and written on the cloud are the words - I am calm and I am confident - and that's exactly how you feel now.

The letters of the words are written in sparkling, glittery dust - and when you see those words on the cloud in your mind - you can allow those words to sprinkle down upon you - for you are calm and you are confident - and so relaxed.

In a moment or two I'm going to count you up to normal conscious awareness - and as you return to the here and now - bring those feelings back with you and let them remain in your mind - accessible whenever you need to feel calm and confident - and so relaxed.

One - you're coming slowly back - two - feeling those wonderful feelings now - growing stronger - three - nearly back - four - eyelids beginning to flicker and five - eyes open and wide awake.

12.3. Progressive Muscle Relaxation Script

There are different styles of progressive relaxation techniques. With some styles you tense a muscle group before you relax that muscle. Personally I never cared for that technique but you can add it to the below relaxation script if that style works for you.

Release the weight of your body into the support of the floor/bed.

Notice how your back makes contact with the support of the floor/bed.

Relax the back of your legs....the back of your hips....your lower back, middle back, and upper back. Feel the weight and relaxation of the back of your body sinking through the floor/bed.

Relax the back of your shoulders / the back of your arms / the back of your neck / and the back of your head. Wiggle and make any adjustments needed to relax the back of your body into the ground more fully. Melt into the support of the floor/bed completely.

Now, notice the weight of your body. Notice the weight of your legs, as they rest on the floor. Let your legs be heavy. Let your thighs, feet and toes relax. Release, relax, let go of them completely. Let your legs drift and float and now forget about them.

Notice the weight of your hips and pelvis, as they rest on the floor/bed. Let the weight of your pelvis sink into the floor/bed.

Notice the weight of your rib cage. Let the back ribs melt into the floor/bed. Feel your abdomen expand with each inhalation. As you exhale, let the belly fully contract. Like a giant balloon inflating and completely deflating.

Relaxing deeper with each deep breath.

Notice the weight of your shoulders and arms, as they rest on the floor/bed. Let your arms be so heavy that they sink through the floor/bed. Then release them completely.

Let go. Let them drift and float away and then forget about them.

Notice the weight of your head, as it rests on the floor/bed. Let the head be heavy. Feel your neck and throat release and relax.

Relax the muscles of your face / relax your eyes and eyelids / your cheeks melt into relaxation / release, relax, let go of your jaw / your forehead and eyebrows smooth and relaxed / feel your scalp melt into relaxation. Your whole head and face totally relaxed, released.

Become aware of your breathing. Notice each inhalation relaxing the front of your body, and each exhalation relaxing the whole back of your body. Breathing slow, deep and then let it go.

Breathing the body deeper and deeper into relaxation as you drift and float in peace.

12.4. How to Be Calm in a Stressful Situation

The clock is ticking. Everyone's counting on you. Which wire do you cut? While most of us never have to deal with the life-or-death dilemmas of a bomb squad, everyday situations, such as job interviews, public speaking, and family emergencies, can be every bit as stressful if we're not accustomed to dealing with them. Learning how to remain calm in times of stress will not only make things go more smoothly immediately, it can also, over time, help you lead a healthier, happier life. Here's how to keep your cool when the pressure mounts.

Steps

Identify the cause of your stress. Is your heart pounding because that idiot just cut you off on the freeway, or is it because of that presentation you have to give to your boss this afternoon? Think for a moment and try to figure out what's really bothering you.

Choose your response. Even if you're powerless to change your stressor, you have the power to choose how you'll respond to it. The appropriate response to stress should depend on what's causing it: you can either shake off your stress (ignore it and let it go immediately) or face it head-on. In order to choose your response - ask yourself some questions.

Does it matter? Yeah, it's all small stuff, but some stuff is smaller than others. Consider how long the stressor will impact you if properly handled. That idiot driver will be gone in a moment if you just let him keep speeding down the road, but the death of a loved one may affect you for years.

How much control do you have over the situation? You can't control the rain that's ruining your wedding, but you can control how well you do on your algebra exam tomorrow.

Is the stressor in the past, present, or future? You can't change the past, but you can react to the present and prepare for the future. Shake off the past.

Shake it off. If a situation is beyond your control, or if it just isn't that important, stop worrying about it. Easier said than done? Just do it.

Inhale deeply and slowly through your nose. Hold each breath for 3-4 seconds, and then exhale slowly through your mouth. Repeat this breathing pattern several times.

Think about something else. Get your mind off the stress by thinking about something that makes you happy, such as your kids or spouse (provided they're not the cause of the current stress), or by concentrating about the things you have planned for the day.

Visualize relaxing things, such as a deserted island or a country road. Close your eyes and try to picture even minor details about the imaginary place, and you can put yourself in that situation instead of the one you're in.

Get away from the cause of the stress. If you can physically escape the stress trigger, do so. Leave the room or pull off the road for a moment to put things in perspective.

Get some exercise. Whether you go for a run, do callisthenics, do yoga, or lift weights, 10-20 minutes of physical exercise can relax you even when nothing else can. Getting plenty of exercise also helps you react better to stress in the long run.

Face your stressor head-on. Stress about future events is mostly caused by fear, and stress over things in the present is usually caused by a feeling of powerlessness. If you can change the outcome of a situation that matters to you, the quickest way to overcome that fear or to empower yourself is to take action as quickly as possible. The steps below will help you. If you feel paralyzed, use the steps above to relax and temporarily distance yourself from the situation just long enough to be able to see it clearly.

Realize that getting stressed is not going to resolve the situation. Sitting around worrying is a good way to procrastinate, but procrastinating will only prolong or intensify the stress.

Make a plan. Sometimes you can resolve a stressful situation right away with one action, but often you'll need several steps, perhaps over a long period. Write out a plan with attainable goals and a timeline for reaching those goals.

Take one step at a time. A complex problem can be overwhelming, even when you've got your plan mapped out, but remember: the journey of a thousand miles begins with one step. Just focus on one small goal at a time.

Trust yourself. If people trust you to do something important, they probably have a reason for doing so.

Be realistic. If you continue to experience stress because no matter how hard you try you can't take the steps quickly enough, you probably haven't set realistic goals. In a culture that values a can-do attitude, it can be hard to accept that sometimes you can't do something, at least not within a given period of time. If that's the case, revise your timeline or lower your expectations. If you can't do that, the situation qualifies as one which you can't control. Learn from you experience, but let it go.

Tips

Facing your stress head-on **and** doing something about your stressor is really just a way to shake off stress about a situation that you cannot or should not ignore. Once you've resolved the underlying problem, you can shake off the stress because it no longer matters.

Many stressful situations are avoidable. If you prepare ahead of time for important events and make contingency plans, you may not have to cope with as much stress later. An ounce of prevention is worth a pound of cure.

Chew gum. It has been shown that the action of chewing can reduce stress; this is why many people who are under constant stress tend to overeat. Chewing gum is a healthier alternative if this method works for you.

Focus on someone else who is in the same situation as you and try to tune in to that person's calm. Remember that if he or she isn't nervous, you probably don't have to be.

If physically able, hit something. Punch a pillow, kick the couch, squeeze the heck out of a stuffed toy, etc. You'd be surprised at how quickly physical venting can reduce stress.

If you experience chronic stress - if you find yourself frequently breaking down in tears, rapidly gaining or losing weight, or experiencing a diminished sex drive - see a doctor about your symptoms. You may have an anxiety disorder or other illness.

Warnings

Inappropriate reactions to stress or an inability to cope with stress can shave years off your life.

Getting in the habit of hitting things while angry might make you a violent/aggressive person. It's better to defuse your anger than to try to take it out on other people or things. Never hit a person or other living thing, and make sure that whatever inanimate object you hit won't hurt you.

Don't self-medicate. Alcohol and drugs may provide a temporary escape, but your problems will be waiting for you when you get back to reality.

See a health professional immediately if you experience chest pain or dizziness.

12.5. How to Create A Home Spa Experience Without Spending A Fortune

Here are some home spa tips that will make you look and feel like a million bucks. Squeeze a few more minutes into your daily routine for them, and become happier and fantastically refreshed!

Steps

Slow down. Take in the experience of an everyday activity that you usually fly through, such as a bath or shower, listening to a favourite song, or even getting dressed in a favourite outfit. Remember why each thing is special to you.

Use an essential oil compress to refresh and energize.

Shower with a gentle, scented gel and a body scrubber. There are many kinds of scrubbers - choose one that exfoliates and stimulates your circulation without making you feel like you've just been rubbed by a cheese grater.

Soak in a bath. Add 5 to 10 drops of an essential oil to bath salts.

Be nice to yourself. These are your precious rejuvenating moments. Take your time.

Be gentle when washing your body or face. Scrubbing too hard or too vigorously can advance signs of ageing in the skin.

Pamper your hair, which takes a beating both indoors and outdoors, all day long. Use a hot oil or deep conditioning treatment and spend the wait time reading a book in the tub!

Replenish lost moisture to your skin and hair by taking two tablespoons of organic flaxseed oil twice a day. You'll get rid of dry skin and combat wrinkles.

Treat your fabulous face like royalty. The skin on your face is thinner and more fragile than the rest of your body. Avoid extremely hot water, harsh soaps or any drying cleansers. Wash with gentle cleansers that don't dry out your skin, and always rub gently as you wash. Moisturise.

Tone and plump the skin on your face by putting an ice cube into a plastic bag, and rubbing it gently all over your face for a couple of minutes.

Rejuvenate from the inside as well. Drink 8 to 10 glasses of water every day.

Eat lots of whole foods, green vegetables, fresh fruits, grains, nuts and lean protein to reduce inflammation, replenish moisture and bring back a youthful glow.

Take 3 full, deep breaths from your abdomen (keep your shoulders still) to complete your simple happy essential home spa experience.

Tips

The benefits and joy you experience during your at home spa day will be more coloured by your desire and your intentions than any fancy, expensive products you can buy.

Be mindful, set your intentions and gradually transition in to or out of your work day.

12.6. How to De-Stress Yourself

Life comes at you in all directions. To remain positive, you must tap into your inner self.

Steps

Wake up every day with a smile on your face.

Whatever happened yesterday, keep it there. Today is a new day. A new day is a new challenge and deserves a new approach. Try doing things a little differently each day.

Get some alone time. If you spend your whole day surrounded by people, you are going to end up stressed. Spend some time in your bedroom reading a book.

Start and complete everything you do. Don't do things half-assed.

Make peace with yourself and your past. If you hurt a person's feelings yesterday, apologize to them today. If you hold onto guilt and anger, you will live a stressed and miserable life.

Learn to forgive, rather than forget.

Try going on a walk for a few minutes. The fresh air and alone time gives you time to think and cool off.

Put on some music you love, draw a warm bubble bath, grab a bar of chocolate, and grab a good, funny book. Stay in as long as you want. Chances are you'll come out in a great mood.

Listen to running water.

Something you can also do is gently massage your sides from your armpits down to your hips with your fingernails.

Feel the air around you. Let it flow gently around you and engulf you. Feel it blow through your hands. This works best when you're outside.

Tips

Whenever you are faced with a stressful situation always remember that there is another way to handle things.

Being alone for 5-15 minutes can really make your stress disappear. It allows your body and mind to calm down.

If your creative 'bug' is to paint or sew, complete the task. It will make you feel proud of yourself. That gives you new confidence.

Learn to breathe properly. The best way is to inhale from the pit of your stomach and then slowly exhale through your nose.

Repeat a mantra like, "I feel relaxed and wonderful." Repeat it as many times as necessary.

Avoid being critical towards yourself. It brings your good mood down, which could also lead to you being a pessimist about everything.

There is a lesson to be learned in everything.

Warnings

If being stressed is making you lean towards drugs or alcohol, remember that this is just a quick fix and ultimately solves nothing.

If stress is starting to affect your life, consider talking to a professional.

12.7. How to Have a Day of Relaxation (for Women)

Every woman needs one of these at least once in their lifetime, why not now? So get someone to take the kids for a few hours, (unless you don't have any) and take some time for a day of relaxation!

Steps

Rent a great chick-flick, drama, or anything that you enjoy.

Grab a pair of sweatpants, and a t-shirt, and put them in your bathroom. Collect any CDs that you might have, that are relaxing or soothing. Start filling up your bath tub, and if you have any, and add some lightly scented bubble bath. Before you get in, bring CD player in, and put in a CD of your choice (one of the ones that you collected).

Stay in the bathtub for as long as you need. Upon getting out, change into the sweatpants and t-shirt, so you can be comfy.

Switch on your TV and pop in your movie of choice. While the previews are playing, pop some popcorn, or gather some snacks.

Gather up any nail-polish supplies you have, and start the movie. While watching it, paint your nails and/or toenails, and have a good cry, laugh, or gawk in suspense.

After the movie, change into a pair of pyjamas, and get a good night's rest.

Tips

Don't feel like renting a movie? Check to see if any good movies are on TV, or watch a favourite movie that you own!

You can replace these clothes items with anything you want, as long as it's comfortable. Pyjamas work fine too, if you're doing this later in the day.

If you have a CD player near your bathroom, put the CD in there, and turn it up so you can hear it. This may be safer than actually having it in your bathroom.

If you don't have bubble bath, shower/bath gel or bar soap work great too.

Snack types can vary, so if you prefer veggies and dip, over chips and popcorn, go for it! This is your day, after all!

If you want, invite a few friends over for watching the movie, so you can have fun together.

I would suggest doing this on the weekend (Saturday or Sunday), or in the evening.

You can check "How to Make Your Own Bath Salts" if you would like to use bath salts instead!

This guide was intended for women, because men may not find it very relaxing to watch a chick-flick (boring yes, relaxing, no) or use bubble bath. But, if you're a man and find these things relaxing, these steps will probably work for you, too.

Alternatives

Meditation: Try meditating, or resting quietly with the goal of completely clearing your mind. You will inevitably start to think about something, just notice that, acknowledge it, and gently bring yourself back to a silent mind. Whatever you were thinking of will still be there when you leave this state, but putting it down for a moment, 5 minutes, or an hour, will re-energize your mind and help you to deal with any task.

Yoga: Some simple stretching of the body can do wonders to relax muscle tension as well as mental tension.

Warnings

As the tag on most CD players imply, it is not safe to operate the CD player while your hands are wet. Do not attempt.

Read the bottles on all products you are going to use before you use them, as you could be allergic to the ingredients.

12.8. How to Relax

Stress has negative consequences to both your health and your relationships. The way to stay healthy and happy is to learn how to relax.

Steps

Begin eating a healthy diet - start today! Sugar and caffeine are your enemies, as they both cause severe ups and downs, upsetting your body's ability to regulate energy. Instead of sugary, carbohydrate loaded snacks (like cookies or granola bars), eat fresh fruits and whole grain breads or crackers (sugar-free). Make sure you get plenty of protein, like that found in chicken, lean beef, whole grains, and low-fat dairy.

When you feel overwhelmed, find a quiet place. Even the stall of a bathroom will work if you have no other place to go. Once in a quiet place, close your eyes and picture your own personal paradise. Put yourself there and imagine the setting. What do you see around you? Is there a breeze? What do you hear - birds? Waves? Water? Imagine yourself thoroughly enjoying every moment here in your special place.

Breathe. Inhale deeply, counting to five, then exhale slowly, counting to five. Do this ten times.

When you return to work (or school), pick one task, only one and focus on it. When it is finished, pick the next one. Do not allow yourself to think about all the other millions of things you have to do. Think about the task at hand only, until you have to set it aside and work on something else.

Avoid people who walk around with their 'hair on fire'. Stress can be contagious, so avoid transmitters.

If you are engaging in behaviours that make you feel guilty, stop! Seek help from a professional if necessary, but don't allow destructive behaviour to sabotage your life and your health. Guilt is a potent source of stress, so get rid of the source of guilt by behaving yourself.

Exercise every day. You don't need to work out like a body builder or celebrity. At least twenty minutes (or more, if you like) every day of moderate activity, like walking or bike-riding, is the best known, scientifically proven way to significantly reduce stress. Walk on a treadmill every day for twenty minutes, take the stairs instead of the elevator, and park a little further away from the entrance to stores. You will be amazed at how much easier you overcome stress when you exercise regularly.

Learn to prioritize. Make a list, every single day, of what you must accomplish that day. Put the most important things at the top and list every task in descending order of importance. Learn to be proactive and take care of things before they become a problem, then your time will be more productive and you will feel less stress.

Tips

Drink tea instead of coffee.

Smile and laugh. Laughing releases endorphins, which fight stress, help you relax, and remind you that life is about more than work. Make it a point to smile more, even if it feels strange at first.

When you first start cutting sugar from your diet you will crave it terribly. Be strong! After a couple of days the cravings will subside and you will notice (already) how much better you feel.

Take a multi-vitamin, some vitamins help relieve stress.

Warnings

Avoid *toxic* people! People who try to guilt you into doing things, or tell you you're not good enough, are people you should spend minimal time with (yes, even if they are family). Your life and health are YOUR responsibility.

If stress is causing serious problems such as ulcers, headaches, or other symptoms, seek help from a doctor.

If you feel the need to drink alcohol or use drugs to "escape" from your stress, please seek professional help IMMEDIATELY.

13. Final Words

Well done. You have now reached the end of this book.

I hope it has given you an insight of how you too can reduce your stress and become more relaxed in this hectic world, ready to help not just yourself, but maybe others too.

Wishing you well on your journey to a happier and more fulfilling life.

Here's a list of my other books:

How to grow your Therapy Business

How to build a high income business
as a Professional Speaker

**Visit my website for great business
related blogs**